Courage to Live Your Dream

La Wanna Parker

DEDICATION

To My Husband, Robert Parker, and My Sons, Robert Jr., Tamboura, Yusef, Arian Sr., My Grandson I Raised, Arian Jr., My Niece, Sherika, All My Grand and Great Grandchildren. You Mean The World To Me. To My Mom and Dad. I wish you were here with me now.

To my sister Nora Jackson. who has always supported and believed in me even when I stubbled along the way. She has always been there for me and lifted me up when I started to fall. I love you, Sis! When you are ready to move forward, I will be there for you as well. I love you and I am so proud of you and all you have accomplished.

My greatest thanks, love, gratitude, and appreciation goes to my Heavenly Father and my Lord Jesus Christ for their total love and support through all things. Thank you for reminding me you have always been with me, just waiting for me to notice.

CONTENTS

	Acknowledgments	i
1	How it Began	Pg #1
2	The Journey Starts	Pg #6
3	What Now?	Pg #12
4	Depression	Pg #19
5	Survivor	Pg #26
6	Assessment	Pg #30
7	Accept	Pg #34
8	Embrace	Pg #38
9	Act	Pg #41
10	Change	Pg #43
	Bonus Information	Pg #54

ACKNOWLEDGMENTS

To Janie D. Who took a chance in supporting a stranger out of the goodness of her heart, Susan S. Who said she saw something special in my spirit that moved her, Christy I. Who kept telling me I could do it, Tonya P. Who told me I had it in me, Tony W. Who said just do it, Tonya H. Who kept telling I could it, Katrina S. Who wanted to know what was stopping me, Caterina R. Who believed I had great mastery in me, Brian B. Who told me from day one I could do it, Gary and Chuck Who always encouraged me, Sheya S. Who started me down this road and had patience with me, Carla P. Who volunteered to help in any way she could, Kim N., who stroked my ego, Pastors Juanita M. and Chyrell E. Who both guided me in the right direction for my life, and a special thank you to Raven, the Show Maven, Who kept at me until she got me on the radio. Thank you all for your love, friendship, and support.

Chapter 1
How it Began

"Nothing is so painful to the human mind as a great and sudden change." — Mary Shelley, Frankenstein

I never gave any real thought to getting older. Maybe because I never felt like I was getting older. My thoughts changed. I know that I am no longer a twenty-something and I have no desire to go back in time to be that age again. I love being the age that I am at every given moment I am alive.

A few years ago, I realized that every day I lived was a gift from God. I started thanking God every morning for allowing me to wake up to a new day and new experiences.

It is strange. I have always believed in God and tried to live my life in a way so that others would know without me saying a word, that I was a God-fearing child. However, my faith and trust were lacking. Perhaps, that is why my life changed; I had come to a point in which I began to question my own existence. What purpose did I serve?

I thought I had at least three to five years of employment left before I would have to retire. However, the day came when I found I had joined the ranks of the unemployed. Unfortunately, I was not prepared to take that plunge yet. Are any of us ever ready for that?

The first few months, were not so bad. I had a few dollars saved, I had applied for Social Security, and I believed that I would be receiving unemployment. So, I would get up when I wanted, even though I still woke at 6 a.m. every morning. I could watch what I wanted on TV and read as much as I wanted in between taking care of my mother and my husband.

My mother had lost most of her vision and could only make out dark shapes. She needed me to do the things she could no longer do for herself. My husband was still having his good and bad days from radiation and chemo therapy and there were days when it was not easy to be around either one.

But then, reality set in. Our financial situation had changed drastically. I was turned down for unemployment. The money I thought would be there for emergencies, would last at best two to three years, if I was careful with spending. So, I had two major problems: 1.) I needed to go back to work; 2.) I was considered too old to hire. No one was interested in hiring a senior citizen, especially one who wanted to work part-time so she could take care of her personal family responsibilities

After weeks of no success at finding a job, another problem popped up, I realized I didn't want to work for another company. I had spent fifty years working for companies with nothing to show for it. I wanted something of my own, but what?

My problem? What did I want to do? What could I do? There are so many things I have a genuine interest in, but non-I have a real do or die passion for, unless it's reading my romance stories. I will never be too old to enjoy my romance stories. I heard a coach say, "I am a jack of all trades and master of several." That was my problem!

There were many times I would go into the bathroom and cry. I would pray because I didn't know what else to do. I asked God if there was something He had for me to do. Everyone speaks of their God given purpose, but after weeks of praying, I still had no idea what my purpose was or what I should put my efforts into. I knew God was there and heard my prayers, but like so many people, I was getting impatient.

I even became jealous of my husband because things were going well for him and I resented having to ask him for money. I was used to having my own money and taking care of my own responsibilities. Now, I needed help and I didn't know how to humble myself and ask for it. I was so busy feeling sorry for myself, I almost missed the small crack in the door that the Lord had opened for me to begin my journey.

Chapter 2
THE JOURNEY BEGINS

*Life is not what it's supposed to be. It's what it is.
The way you cope with it is what makes the
difference.* - Virginia Satir

My journey began when a friend was
to be a guest speaker at a "Words Have
Power" Summit and asked me to come
support him. Now he is a very popular
person, very well liked, and I knew for a fact
he had invited quite a few people to attend
his speaking engagement. So, I started
thinking, "He doesn't need me there. He
probably won't even notice if I don't show
up." I know, selfish on my part. I told you I

was feeling sorry for myself and quite selfish.

I didn't understand why my life had chosen to go in a negative direction. I kept asking God why this was happening. I didn't know what to do or who else to ask for help.

The day of the program, I was feeling depressed. My mom had spent the morning complaining about the loss of her vision. It bothered me that she still was not appreciative of all God had given her when I was failing at everything so badly. My mom had children who loved and respected her. God had provided her with an unexpected monthly income, so she did not have to worry about bills and how she was to purchase groceries. He even provided her with the money to pay off her house.

My mom was a strong woman; stronger than even she realized. My Mother was the kind of woman who could not be detoured once she had set her mind on what she wanted to accomplish. She didn't have much in the way of clothes, but she dressed the best she could and took care of herself and us. The neighbors thought she was uppity when she enrolled herself in night school. Some said she thought she was better than they were because the Housing Authority in the project we lived in, offered her a part time job working in the toy loan center. What little money they paid decreased what she owed for rent. My Mother did not concern herself with what others said or thought about her. She worked hard to make something of herself.

My Mother set four goals for herself and she never gave up believing she would have her dream. Her goals were to 1) have a car, 2) her own home, 3) work for the Post Office, and 4) have money in the bank. Personally, I didn't see how this was going to happen! We were on welfare and my mother had only an eighth-grade education.

Years passed with her still talking about these dreams. Three of us became adults and moved out and she continued to believe in her dreams. Things changed when my brother who had become a marine and was sent either across country or overseas. Honestly, I don't remember which. My brother had a car and decided to give it to my mother! This apparently was what God was waiting to happen because within a few weeks, all those test my mother took for the Post Office paid off. She finally got the call she had been waiting for and became a postal worker.

The other two dreams became a piece of cake. She saved her money and when they built new homes in the Compton area, she bought a brand-new home and still had money in the bank. We were all wildly happy for her, but that wasn't all. When she retired, she bought another new home in a city hundreds of miles away. My mother was a **strong** woman and she **never** gave up on her dreams.

Now! Why did I share that story? To tell you 1) hold to your dreams, 2) no matter what the circumstances or obstacles facing you, you must continue to work toward your dream, and 3) I'm not my mother!

I am a witness to my mothers' dreams becoming a reality. I can bare testimony that trusting in God and holding onto her faith, that He would deliver kept her going. She believed, and it became her reality.

So, what happened to me? I had it too easy. I didn't have her struggles, but I thought I knew how to handle it if I ever had to go through anything like she did. I guess I was too cocky and didn't think I would have to worry about something like that happening to me. I thought I had everything under control only to find out I couldn't have been further from the truth.

So, when I returned home after taking care of my mothers' needs, and that of my sister who was little more than a child herself, I was not going to this event. After all, my friend had enough people who would be attending the event to support him. He wouldn't even know I was not there.

I kept telling myself that right up to an hour before the program, when I heard a whisper in my ear, "you need to go". I don't know where the voice came from. I choose to believe it was the voice of God speaking to me. At any rate, I jumped up and gave myself a quick "H" bath and put on a touch of makeup and drove as quickly as I could to the program. I was about 15 minutes late, but the program still had not started. It was as if they were waiting for me to arrive. So, I visited with some of the vendors and asked questions while waiting for the program to start.

The speakers were good, but I was thinking, "How does any of this help me?" I had not experienced the horrific things they were sharing and overcame. Don't get me wrong, I thought it admirable what they had overcome and how they turned their lives around and were doing wonderful things. Only, I hadn't experienced those types of things. So, where did I fit in?

Chapter 3
WHAT NOW?
Be happy for this moment. This moment is your life.
- Anonymous

As I sat there during intermission feeling sorry for myself...again. A young woman I had met earlier, came over and said she had someone she wanted me to meet because she felt compelled to introduce us and the woman had made an enormous difference in her life. I was introduced to Sheya Chisenga, who would later become a good friend and coach.

She helped me to see that I may not have had those types of horrific experiences in life, but the things I had experienced had made me who I am, and I needed to share that with others who may feel as I did. Sometimes, we believe because we have not had anything horrible happen in our lives, we don't matter and what we have to say doesn't mean anything to others.

I have come to realize it does matter and there are others who need to hear what we have experienced. My trials and tribulations may not have been horrific, but they made me who I am today.

My father left us when I was about nine, but I knew he loved me and my siblings. My mom had six children with my father and later had two more. She could have dumped us on the state, but she took care of us the best she could with what she had. My parents never mistreated us, but I was the one they both confided in when they needed to talk. I knew both sides of the story of their divorce.

Other than growing up and often being told I could not have the dreams I wanted from well-meaning friends and relatives, being hungry, and feeling the burden of responsibility for my mother and siblings, I had it pretty good compared to so many stories I have heard over the years. One of my best friends had an abusive father; he was always beating on his kids and wife. My friend often spoke of leaving home as soon as she turned eighteen. She did leave home, but seven years later she passed away. I never learned the details behind her death, only she left behind two children.

I attended Sheya's workshops and later the workshops of others. I realized, I enjoyed being around people who were going after their dreams. It helped me to remember some of the dreams I had as a child. There were two I often thought of but never attempted to do anything about.

I grew up in the fifties and early sixties when you were put down by others for reaching beyond what the community thought you capable of achieving. I wanted to learn to speak before people; however, I was the quiet shy girl who was afraid to speak up. My other dream was to write a book someday. The kids thought it funny. What would I write about and who would be interested? To make matters worse, I created a diary out of a tablet. I wrote my thoughts and feelings there and kept it hidden under the mattress.

Unfortunately, one of my sisters found it and thought it would be funny to share with the other kids. I was never so humiliated as when the others laughed at some of the things I had written there. It was the excuse I needed to put away my writing and not attempt to even write a letter for years.

You are probably wondering if I did anything about those two dreams? Well, yes! I joined *Toastmasters* and learned to speak before club members and later, at workshops and conferences. I highly recommend *Toastmasters* for anyone who must lead a meeting or speak before any group.

The fact that you are reading this book, tells you I must have done something to get me to write again. Yes! I wrote this book. These are my words. I decided I wanted to write bad enough to do something about it and if no one was interested in reading my work, then so be it.

I took an online writing class and later entered a short story contest. *Wonder of Wonders!* My story and nine other stories were selected as winners and published in an anthology in Australia called *"Stories One."* So now, I can call myself an international author and contest winner. Since then I have written a chapter in three other books and wrote a goals journal.

However, I digress from my purpose in writing this book. You see, despite my mothers' accomplishments and my own successes in life, when trouble hit I wasn't prepared to handle it and it was tearing me apart. For the first time, I had a situation I had no idea how to handle and I was becoming more depressed every day.

In fact, I became so depressed that I started thinking there was no reason for being here, and even pondered on the idea of suicide. It didn't go beyond that and only for a few seconds. I might have been down, but I am still a survivor.

At this point in my life, everything that could go wrong, went wrong. There are three reasons I did not act on that suicide thought; 1) I do believe in God and I knew that was not an option; 2) I am a strong woman myself and I was not going to give into a one way trip, and 3) God put Sheya in my life and I started to notice slight changes as I saw the possibilities before me.

However, if you expect me to say things changed overnight, I'm going to disappoint you. I enjoyed being with people who were doing things with their lives, but I had recaptured the lack of self-confidence from my youth and the failures I experienced in recent years and now had a tight grip on me. It was a difficult thing to let go of all those negative thoughts that had such a tight strangle hold on me.

Chapter 4
DEPRESSION

"I don't want to see anyone. I lie in the bedroom with the curtains drawn and nothingness washing over me like a sluggish wave. Whatever is happening to me is my own fault. I have done something wrong, something so huge I can't even see it, something that's drowning me. I am inadequate and stupid, without worth. I might as well be dead." – Margaret Atwood, *Cat's Eye*

I never thought of myself as someone who would become depressed. I didn't realize I was depressed about anything because I continued functioning with the day to day ritual of living.

I now realize it started with the death of my first-born son. I was devastated, but I don't think anyone knew it. I happened to hear my husband telling one of our friends, "Oh, I wouldn't worry about La Wanna. She can handle anything. She's ok."

I silently walked away from the conversation and said nothing. Inside I was burning up with anger, hurt, and resentment. How dare anyone think I was alright when I had just buried my baby! He wasn't really a baby. He had only been twenty-three for twenty-three days when he died in a car accident. He had spent five years in the Army and was so proud to be a member of the 82nd Airborne Special Forces Rangers Unit and engaged to get married. He had his whole life before him and I felt as if my heart had been ripped from my body.

I tried to find a quiet place to think about what I had overheard to no avail. I was hurting from the loss of my son and no one seemed to realize it was my son who had died. They were counting on me to console them.

That was the start of depression for me. I didn't know it at the time because I had three other sons, a niece, and later, a grandson who needed me to be there for them.

It was several months after losing my job that I started to realize something was happening and it wasn't good. Negative thoughts were choking the life out of me. My money was running low, so I swallowed my pride and asked my former employer if I could apply for unemployment since they had called me in a few times to help when they were shorthanded, but it had been several weeks since the last call and I was concerned about my finances.

They gave me the ok, but the Unemployment Office turned me down. I appealed it, but they still denied me.

I didn't know what to do. I had put in several applications with no success. Not even an interview or a call or letter to say, "No thanks." I knew it had to be my age. At least that's what I thought was the reason. My real problem, I was competing against college students and everyone else looking for a job. My age may have been a small factor, but they could hire someone else with less experience for less money.

So, when I went to the "Words Have Power Speaker's Summit," I was feeling down in the dumps and feeling sorry for myself. After meeting Sheya, she invited me to attend an intro meeting she was having. I was ready to try anything to get pass the feeling of worthlessness I was experiencing.

I started attending workshops and they were motivational and inspirational because I heard women with real deep problems speak of how they were overcoming their situations and moving on with their lives. They were not sitting around feeling sorry for themselves. They were doing something about their situation. I was beginning to realize, maybe I could find something to do and start a new career.

A few short months later, I went to my mother's home as I did every day to help her and do her grocery shopping. My mother was sitting on the couch and did not answer when I spoke to her. I asked a question and it dawned on me that she was not responding to me. At first, I thought she was sleeping.

I walked over to shake her on the shoulders. Still no answer or response even though I raised my voice. I knew something was wrong now, because my mother has always been a light sleeper.

I touched her neck and it felt cool to the touch and no pulse. I put my head to her chest and I couldn't hear or feel a heartbeat. I ran to get a mirror out of her bedroom and held it under her nose. Nothing! I called 911 and they directed me to give her CPR until the paramedics arrive.

The paramedics arrived and took over giving her CPR. After three or four minutes of trying to resuscitate her, the paramedics pronounce her dead.

The year before I lost my job, I had to make the awful decision to take my dad off life support because the family he had raised all those years after leaving us couldn't be bothered.

I hurt for him because none of them was there and I hurt for myself because I had to be the one to make the decision. I spoke with my dad for twenty minutes and then prayed over him for both of us before giving the doctors permission to release him.

Now my mother was gone and once again I was put in the position of having to make decisions I wasn't ready for. I handled it, but I knew something was wrong. I still laugh, smile, and did all that was expected of me, but I knew deep inside that I was beginning to really struggle with myself.

But things began to change even more and for the worst. My money had run out and I only had social security for my financial needs. In trying to help a family member, I got myself in deeper financial trouble. With every decision I made, it turned out wrong and I found the hole I had dug was getting deeper and the despair I was feeling was becoming more than I could tolerate. I felt alone, isolated, and I began to feel my prayers for help were being ignored.

Chapter 5
Survivor

"Your fear is 100% dependent on you for its survival." —Steve Maraboli, <u>Life, the Truth, and Being Free</u>

I have never felt so lost and worthless as I had started to feel. Nothing was going the way it was supposed to. The money I had should have lasted longer, but I decided to pay off the balance I owed on the house. That didn't make things better. They were worse. I had cut into the money I had saved for emergencies and possible trips down to a few hundred dollars and now, I had no backup for emergencies.

I said I was a survivor and I believe I am. I have survived two rapes, one at knife point, the other with a gun in my face, two threats on my life and an ex-boyfriend, who tried to get me to become a prostitute.

I lost my first born-son and two months later, my grandmother. In the last few years since then, I have lost several good friends, my father-in-law, three aunts, my sister, two uncles, my mother-in-law, my father, two brothers-in-law, two cousin-in-law, and my mother. Yes! I am still trying to be strong for everyone.

Once, I was driving on a lonely highway with no music or radio to entertain me, and I believe I closed my eyes for a second, came to myself and slammed on the brakes of my car. I ended up on the other side of the highway, facing the direction I had come from with two completely busted tires. But I was unharmed.

I have been rear-ended twice while sitting at a red light, and deliberately sideswiped on an empty highway. My car was hit so hard the insurance company paid it off. Another time, I was driving when someone decided they wanted to move between me and the car behind me. Either the person miscalculated the distance between our two cars and the speed of the car behind me or the car behind me was not going to let them in. This resulted in the car behind me slamming into the car that was attempting to get in between us, and that car slammed into my car.

Again, I was unhurt. Finally, I was driving on my way to work, when someone in opposing traffic thought he could make a left turn and complete it before I got to the intersection; he was wrong. I slammed on my brakes. I think he did too, but he also slammed into my door so hard it pushed my door in on me and my left leg took the full impact causing it to swell so bad, I could not stand the slightest touch to my leg and foot. My leg and foot were almost double their original size.

Other than that, I was blessed to be unharmed, although my doctor insisted I wear a neck brace for a few weeks just in case and I had to go to a chiropractor for several weeks.

All these things tell me I am a survivor. God has plans for me. However, either he hasn't told me what it is he wants me to do, or I am not seeing it because it's something I don't want to do. You know, we want to do something really big and glamourous and maybe have people see us as something special. I believe that was my problem and why I couldn't see what was before me.

Before you go thinking this a "Oh! Woo is me!" book, it isn't. I am telling you about my dark places and my mindset. Fear, doubt and scarcity came knocking on my door and instead of slamming the door in their face I invited them in and they made themselves at home and refuse to leave.

Meeting Sheya was the beginning steps to get them to leave. Attending the Personal mastery retreat and remembering how important it was to have God in my life gave me the courage to push them out the door. I'll my experiences at the retreat later in this book.

.

Chapter 6
Assessment

"Confront the dark parts of yourself, and work to banish them with illumination and forgiveness. Your willingness to wrestle with your demons will cause your angels to sing." —August Wilson

What do I do about my situation? What now? What do I want to do? If no one wants to hire me and I really don't want to work for another company, what do I do now? Everyone tells me to do the thing I have a great passion for. The only thing I have a great passion for, is reading romance stories, writing, and giving speeches.

Others have told me to think about what people always seem to come to me for. What seems to come so natural to me that people always approach me for that. Well!

People come to me for support, help, advice, suggestions, and encouragement. I have done this for so long for free and the idea of charging, has caused some to think I would be wasting my time.

So, I decided to do an assessment of where I was before, where I am now, and where I want to be in the future. I didn't like much of what I learned about myself, but I believe I have a better understanding of who I am, flaws and all, and I'm ok with that.

How about you? Write an assessment of where your life has been, where it is now, and where you want it to be in the future. Write it on the lines below. Look at your strengths and weaknesses.

Assessment

_____

_____

_____

_____

_____

_____

_____

_____

_____

_____

_____

_____

_____

_____

_____

_____

_____

_____

_____

What did you come up with? It doesn't matter if others think it is silly. Put everything down. Writing it down on paper helps you to see clearly and come to terms with who you are. You don't have to share any of this with anyone. It can be for your eyes only. This is the beginning of learning what you truly want in life.

What's standing in the way of your dreams?

_____

_____

_____

_____

_____

_____

_____

_____

_____

_____

_____

_____

_____

_____

_____

_____

_____

_____

_____

_____

Chapter 7
Accept

"You are imperfect, permanently and inevitably flawed. And you are beautiful." —Amy Bloom

What I have come to terms with is that I am La Wanna Parker. I can't be or do what others are doing because it doesn't work for me and that's ok.

You see, I can continue my reading of romance stories, write whatever strikes me at the time, and give my speeches. These are things I can make money doing, but I also have come to accept that everything in my life has led me to be a supporter, nurturer, helper, and encourager. I have my program to help others to on their path to greatness.

Have you accepted your gifts? Have you discovered your true path? Have you accepted that you are not perfect, but that it is ok? On the line below, write what you have come to accept about who you are.

Acceptance

_____

_____

_____

_____

_____

_____

_____

_____

_____

_____

_____

_____

_____

_____

_____

_____

_____

_____

_____

_____

_____

_____

_____

_____

Don't be discouraged when doing these exercises if nothing comes to mind right away. It took months for me to recognize and accept me as I am. That I was someone worth more than I believed myself to be because of my own limiting beliefs swimming in my head.

You are worth ever so much more than you can imagine. Don't short change yourself by failing to go after your dream. I promise you the journey alone will be well worth any stumbling blocks you come across along the way.

Chapter 8
Embrace

Stop stressing out trying to figure out "how things are supposed to happen," instead allow things to happen. You are on a journey to experience your best life. Do not rob yourself of that because "the experience is the journey and the journey is the experience." (Lewis T. Powell)

When I sat down to assess myself, it was very difficult. I had to look at both my strengths and my weaknesses and I did not like what I saw.

I complained a great deal to myself, that God didn't love me because he was not hearing my prayers or washing away my tears. But that wasn't true. God has always been there for me and I can give you a list of the things he has done for me. I was the one who had moved from him and taken him for granted. I was lacking in faith and trust and without faith, nothing was possible.

I had to accept that failures and wrong decisions I made, were because I did not first turn to God before ploughing ahead and the result was failure after failure.

Now, I have embraced who I was when God was first in my life, who I had become when I forgot and went out on my own, and who I would become now that I recognized I was nothing when I forgot to include Him in all areas of my life.

What have you embraced about your life? Write your answers below. There is no right or wrong way to respond. Just be true to yourself. This is for your eyes only and between you and the higher power you worship.

Embrace

_____
_____
_____
_____
_____
_____
_____
_____
_____
_____
_____
_____
_____
_____
_____
_____
_____
_____
_____
_____
_____
_____
_____
_____
.

Chapter 9
Act

Every morning, Steve Harvey gives listeners a daily dose of knowledge, wisdom, and inspiration with his #FinalThoughts. One morning, he discussed the importance of having a goal versus having a plan. It is important to have goals in our lives, but it is just as important for us to not get "caught up" in the route (or the plan) it takes to get to our goals.

Before you take off after your dream, I want you to write down what that dream is and what resources or information you need before setting up your plans. Use the lines below to write out your dream and why you want it.

Chapter 10
Change

"Incredible change happens in your life when you decide to take control of what you do have power over instead of craving control over what you don't." — Steve Maraboli, Life, the Truth, and Being Free

The process I have described in the previous pages, are what I went through for myself after I returned from a retreat I almost backed out of for financial reasons. I am so glad I did not.

Going on the retreat was the best decision I could have made. The changes in my life happened when I made the decision to go on a Personal Mastery Retreat. On this retreat I met some terrific people.

Janie D. was one of those individuals who came to the rescue of a total stranger. It is not my place to tell her story, but she did something unbelievably great for me and I will never forget it or her. She is the woman on the of this book as we celebrate our success at finishing the program.

The great thing about this five-day retreat, is it challenged us every day to go beyond our comfort zone. I wish I could tell of the challenges. I can only say I discovered I could do things I thought I would never do or have the strength or courage to do because of my fears.

I learned when I faced the fear and did the challenge, I could do it and survive. Then I wondered why I had been afraid. We all had the support of each other, which helped. We encouraged, supported and lifted each other up when it appeared someone would slip. It is amazing what you can do with the support of friends and colleagues.

We were divided up into partners and teams we worked with all week. I made friends I am still in touch with and we continue to support one another. Because of the confidence placed in me, I began to grow my own confidence. I realized that if I could meet the challenges I had at the retreat, then I was the problem that was holding me back.

I was able to confront my hidden fears I didn't realize had and speak openly about them. No, I didn't do an overnight change! It took years for these things to take control of me and it meant I had my work cut out for me. I would have to actively work on my fears, face them, and shove them out of the way because if I held onto them, they had control and that wouldn't do for the new changing me.

It was on this retreat that I knew I had to start making some serious changes in my life. I was scared because I had no idea what I wanted to do, but I began giving it serious thoughts. This has not been an easy process. I have many interests and many things I know I can do that I really enjoy doing! In the end after much thought and going back and forward, I recognized that I like helping and supporting others. Helping them to feel good about themselves. Encouraging them to go after their dreams. Helping them set goals and keeping them accountable.

The members of my retreat team were Lucian, Tom, Cheryl, who is a very special lady and kept us all laughing, Blaine, Janie, and myself. I must mention Susan S., because she sent me a wonderful gift. I was so surprised, and she told me it was because I inspired her and others at my willingness to meet all the challenges presented to us. Andrew told me the same thing and that means so much to me.

You see, I was the oldest female (maybe the oldest) there and I stepped up to the plate even when fear was working against me and kept reminding me of my age. Each time I told it to get behind me because I trusted the man on my right who said I could do it and He would be with me all the way.

I had no idea what we would be doing and it was my first retreat, so I came dressed as I always do. Needless to say, heels and dresses were not the appropriate attire for most of what we did, but I didn't let that stop me. I was just being me and trusting in my Lord.

I am happy and content with the person I am becoming. I say becoming because there is more to me than even I realized and so much I want to do before I go home for my eternal rest. In this book, I have shared the process I used and still use because I am growing and changing all the time. For the better of course!

I have not spoken of coaches or mentors, but I urge you to find one that is a success in whatever field you decide is what you want to do. Everyone should have a coach and mentor. If the coaches and mentors have them and they are successful at what they do, that tells you, you need to get one as well. Just be careful and select the individual who can truly benefit you.

It is my sincere desire that the information I have shared and the steps I provided will help you. They are not perfect, but you must start somewhere, and this is as good a place any. I have made the steps easy and this book a quick read, so you can start right away on the new you.

As I say on my radio show, "New Direction, New Attitude, New You!"

Now that you know what your dream or goal is and why you want it, start planning what you need to do to achieve your dream.

I know you have come up with more than one goal, but for now I want you to work on one.

Here are my seven steps to help you get from where you are to where you want to be:

1. Determine the dream
2. Set the goal to achieve the dream
3. Research what you need to make this a reality
4. Plan small steps to get you to your goal
5. Set a time limit for each step and adjust what you are doing if needed
6. Act. If you don't move to take action, it's only a hobby or wishful dreaming

7. Reward yourself after you achieve each step. Make it a big reward with the completion of the project.

My dream:

_____

_____

My goal:

_____

_____

Type of research needed:

_____

_____

_____

_____

Steps to take:

_____

_____

_____

_____

_____

_____

_____

_____

_____

_____

Time limit:

_____

_____

Action/ start and completion date:

_____

_____

Reward for completion:

_____

_____

Notes:

_____

_____

_____

_____

_____

_____

_____

_____

This is the process I started using for myself. As you become more adept at working your goals, you will come up with a process that works better for you, but this will get you started.

If you have followed along and wrote in this book or in your personal notebook or journal, you have accomplished five steps to help you with your dream. But if you are like me, you wanted to read it first.

Summary:

1. **Survivor**-Despite everything that has happened in your life, you are still here with dreams you want to achieve. God has given you everything you need within you to go after your heart's desire.

2. **Assess**-Take an assessment of who you were, where you are now, and what you want for your future.

3. **Acceptance**-None of us are perfect to our way of thinking. But God made you. Therefore, you are perfect as you are and worthy of any dreams you have. Accept that you have made mistakes, but you have learned from them and are a better and stronger person because you survived.

4. **Embrace**-You are worth more than you know. Embrace who you are and share your story with someone who

needs to hear it. Don't be afraid to go after your dream or to ask for help.

5. **Act**-Write out what you want and why. Your why will keep you going when you hit obstacles along the way. Once you know what you want, do your research to determine what you need to start working on your goal.

This is the process I used to help me find my way. But I am convinced none of this would have worked had I not gone on the retreat and remembered to include God every step of the way. You may come up with other steps that work for you, but until you do, this is a stepping stone to help you get started and it is simple. Don't rush the process. Take as much time as you need for each step.

For some of you, you will do this in a matter of hours, others, it could be days, weeks, or even months. For me, it took months.

I am excited because I have my dreams and what I believe God wants me to do. I am an author, blogger, motivational speaker, an encouragement supporter coach, a companion to seniors who need me as much as I need them, and I still get to read my romance stories.

God gave me the courage I needed to live my dream by first sending Sheya Chisenga into my life then sending me on that retreat and finally urging me to place my trust in Him! Fear, scarcity, and self-doubt were eating me up and I thought God no longer cared for me. When I turned back to God, He reminded me He had never left. He was waiting for me to remember He was there and to place my trust back in Him.

All this is possible because I asked God's forgiveness and accepted him back in my life. I joined a Bible Study group, I read the Bible each day, and I start each day with a prayer thanking God for allowing me to take part in another day and for what He has provided for me (family, friends, health, etc.).

At the end of each day, it is my sincere desire that I have made a difference in at least one person's life. More I hope, but at least one and for those whose lives I have touched, I pray you pass it on and make a difference for others. It's why we are here, to help others. God bless you!

Bonus Information

Always remember…

"It Doesn't Matter Where You Came From. All That Matters Is Where You Are Going."- Brian Tracy

Make it your habit to always look to the future, never dwell on the past. If you live by this thought, you will continue to move toward your goals with success.

My personal secret ingredients to succeed, means you must:

1. Know who you are and what you want
2. Be true to your core values and beliefs
3. Be willing to work hard for what you want
4. Never give up on your dream
5. Be trustworthy and reliable
6. Be willing to help others along the way
7. Be positive and friendly with a happy attitude

You will have well-meaning friends and family members who want to protect you from yourself by suggesting you should go for a smaller dream or not try at all. Always remember, your success or failure is in your hands. You make the decisions on what is important to you. You must have the courage to live your dream. It is waiting for you!

"Think Big And Don't Listen To People Who Tell You It Can't Be Done. Life's Too Short To Think Small."- An Awesome Quote By Tim Ferriss

I will end with a quote from two great men:

"Success is not final, failure is not fatal: it is the courage to continue that counts."
Winston Churchill

John 14:13 And whatsoever ye shall ask in my name, that will I do, that the Father may be glorified in the Son. If ye shall ask any thing in my name, I will do it.

Have a God bless day!

ABOUT THE AUTHOR

La Wanna is a dynamic speaker and is an international award-winning co-author and contest winner.

She is a contributing author of Amazon #1 Best Seller, "Conversations Behind the Mic" with Raven Glover.

La Wanna currently has classes on improving your self-esteem and confidence.

Contact information:

LaWanna Parker
916-587-0800 or 916-238-8847
lawanna@lawannaspeaks.com
http://www.lawannagparker.com

facebook.com/lawannaparker

Made in the USA
Middletown, DE
28 May 2023